Best Keto Bread Cookbook

Quick And Easy Ketogenic Bread Recipes For Weight Loss & Optimal Wellbeing

Crystal Darrow

DEDICATION

To the successful pursuit of a healthy life.

Table of Contents

INTRODUCTION 1

BREAD LOAVES RECIPES 3

    Nut Free Keto Bread 4

    Keto Sandwich Bread.. 5

    Low Carb Banana Bread.. 6

    Easy Chia Bread 7

    Low Carb Yeast Sandwich Bread............................... 8

BREADS ROLLS RECIPES 11

    Cheddar Garlic Fathead Rolls................................. 12

    Keto Bread Rolls.. 13

    Hawaiian Sweet Rolls.. 15

    Keto Dinner Rolls 16

    Keto Fiber Bread Rolls 17

BUNS RECIPES... 19

    Keto Bread Buns 20

    Keto Burger Buns 21

    Dark Bread Buns 22

    Low Carb Cauliflower Burger Buns 23

    Perfect Keto Buns 25

BAGEL RECIPES 27

    Keto Fathead Bagels 28

    Bagel Buns With Yeast 29

    Low-Carb Multi Seed Bagels 30

    Low Carb Cinnamon Sugar Bagels 32

Flavored Bagels...33

PIZZA DOUGH RECIPES 35

Keto Fathead Pizza Doug 36

Yeast Pizza Dough 37

Bacon Fathead Pizza Dough..38

Low carb Fathead Pizza Dough 39

Fat Head Pizza Dough 41

TORTILLA RECIPES..43

Keto Coconut Flour Tortillas 44

Easy Low Carb Tortilla...45

Smoked Paprika Tortilla...46

Keto Vegan Tortilla 47

Pork Rind Tortillas...48

MUFFINS RECIPES 49

Keto Blueberry Muffins 50

Ham And Zucchini Muffins 51

Almond Flour Banana Muffins...52

Low Carb Pumpkin Muffins 53

Cheese Muffins...54

CRACKER RECIPES 57

Low Carb Jalapeño Cheese Crackers 58

Easy Crackers 59

Keto Rosemary Crackers..60

Keto Goldfish Crackers 61

Tasty Crackers..62

BREADSTICKS RECIPES 63

Cauliflower Breadsticks 64

Taco Stuffed Breadsticks 65

Cheesy Zucchini Breadsticks... 66

Low Carb Cauliflower Breadsticks 67

Breadsticks With Sesame Seeds 69

INTRODUCTION

The keto diet has healthy -fat, appropriate -protein, and low-carbohydrate that buns fat and keeps the body in ketosis state. Taking less of carb helps the body to break down excess fats into ketones. Ketones are chemicals in your liver, produced when you don't have enough glucose in your body for energy, so fat is substitute for sugar to supply energy, and this is the best way because too much of high carb foods or sugar causes cravings for more sugary things, your body turns the excess carbs into unwanted fats in the body, and some diseases like; gallbladder disease, respiratory issues, diabetes, obesity and some more.

You may lose some strength at the beginning of your keto diet, this is normal because your body is used to burning carbs for fuel. Symptoms like fatigue, headaches, and sluggishness may occur too, it is called keto-flu, but once fully adapted to keto diet and burning fat for fuel, you have more energy on like before you need to consume more carb for energy but now your body has more fat to work on. These symptoms typically last for three days

The keto diet is not for energy or for weight controlling alone, also used to treat patient with certain medical conditions like cancer, diabetes and sometimes eliminate seizures in some patients. The keto diet helps reduce anxiety, you sleep sounder, controls your appetite, lowers blood pressure, regulates blood sugar level, reduces risk of heart diseases, and lot more. Some yet to be discovered.

For best result, 30–50 grams of carbs is normally the recommended amount to start with. Once you get use to eating "Keto" you can reduce carbs as you like even to 20 grams. But it is up to you and all depends on how fast you can adapt. {For fat 75 percent and protein 20 percent}.

Substituting carbs with keto diet will make you consume less. You won't consume more because the foods are filling. Keto averagely consist of almonds, avocado, eggs, cheese, broccoli, chicken, nuts, salmon, and vegetables. When it comes to protein egg is a great source or protein for keto, ground beef, steaks, salmon, chicken, pork, bacon, hot dogs, fatty fish and some more. For fat and oil it is important you know the quality of the fats you consume {natural and processed one}. Natural polyunsaturated fats can be found from fatty fish, lard, avocados, nuts, egg yolks, grass-fed butter, ghee, coconut butter, cocoa butter, mayonnaise, extra-virgin olive oil and some more. Processed fats should be avoided.

Vegetables are to be consumed more in keto but you should also choose your vegetables wisely because some have high carb. Examples of healthy vegetables for keto diet are: kale, spinach, broccoli, cauliflower, Brussel sprout, cabbage, cauliflower, cucumber, eggplant, fennel, green beans, arugula, asparagus, artichokes and some more. Also on keto diet there re fruits to take, such as Blueberries, Cherries, Cantaloupe, Cranberries, Coconut, Strawberries, Raspberries, Tomatoes, Lemons and limes.

Let's bake!

BREAD LOAVES RECIPES

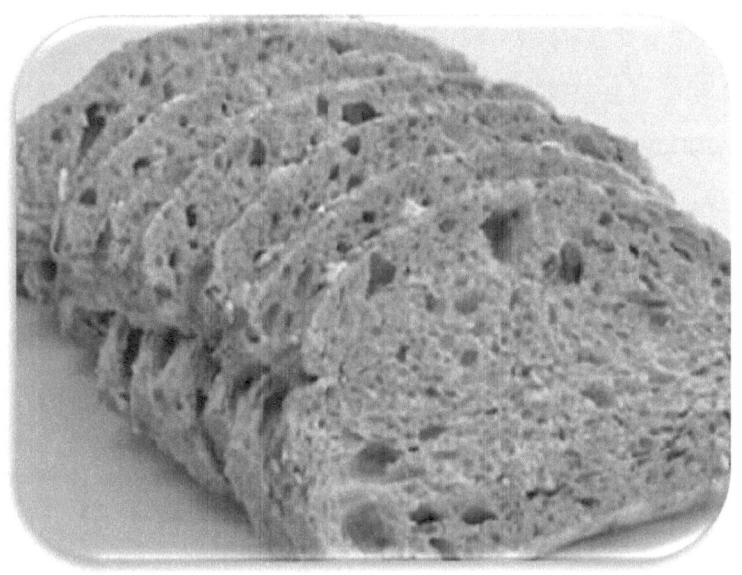

Nut Free Keto Bread

Enjoy a delicious and healthy bread

Prep Time; 10 minutes

Cook Time: 45 minutes

Serves: 12 slices

Ingredients

1/4 cup chia seeds

1/2 cup coconut flour

1/2 cup hemp hearts

1/2 cup golden flax

2 tablespoons psyllium powder

1 cup warm water

2 tablespoons avocado oil

2 tablespoons sweetener

2 teaspoons vinegar

1 teaspoon baking soda

4 eggs

1 teaspoon salt

Directions

1. Turn on oven to 350 degrees, oil loaf pan, blend chia seed, hemp hearts, and golden flax in a blender to powder.

2. Add psyllium powder, baking soda, and coconut flour to the blended seeds and mix well to combine.

3. Add avocado oil, eggs, vinegar, and warm water. Stir thoroughly for about 2 minutes.

4. Use a spatula to put the mixture in the oiled loaf pan, and bake for about 55 minutes in the oven. When ready let it cool before slicing.

5. Enjoy!

Nutrition Information Per- Serving: Calories: 171 kcal; Fat: 12g; Carbohydrates: 8g; Protein: 7g

Keto Sandwich Bread
So healthy and satisfying

Prep Time; 10 minutes

Cook Time; 30 minutes

Serves; 10 slices

Ingredients

1 tablespoon baking powder

2 cups almond flour

1/2 cup almond milk

1/4 cup melted butter

1/4 cup golden flax, blended

4 eggs

1/4 teaspoon salt

Directions

1. Mix flour, baking powder, almond milk, melted butter, golden flax and egg in a bowl.

2. Pour mixture in a bread pan and bake in an oven at 400°F for about 30 minutes.

3. Let it cool before serving. Enjoy!

Nutrition Information Per- Serving: Calories: 255 kcal; Fat: 12.8g; Carbohydrates: 3.5g; Protein: 4.3g

Low Carb Banana Bread
So crunchy! The taste you will like.

Prep Time; 5 minutes

Cook Time; 60 minutes

Serves; 10 slices

Ingredients

3 ripe banana, crushed

3 eggs

2 cups almond flour

1/4 cup olive oil

1 teaspoon baking soda

Sweetener

Directions

1. In a bowl, beat eggs, add crushed banana, olive oil and mix well.

2. In another bowl add almond flour, baking soda, and sweetener. Mix well and add to the first mixture.

3. Spray loaf pan with oil, stir mixture well and pour into pan. Bake for about 60 minutes on oven at 350°F.

4. Enjoy!

Nutrition Information Per- Serving: Calories: 269 kcal; Fat: 22g; Carbohydrates: 15g; Protein: 8g

Easy Chia Bread
So easy! Super tasty!

Prep Time: 5 minutes

Cook Time: 90 minutes

Serves: 3 slices

Ingredients

4 large tablespoon almond flour

1/4 teaspoon mustard powder

1 teaspoon baking powder

2 tablespoon chia seeds, blended

1/4 teaspoon garlic powder

2 eggs

Salt

Pepper

Directions

1. In a bowl, mix thoroughly almond flour, baking powder, garlic powder, blended chia, mustard powder, pepper, and salt.

2. Whisk eggs and add to the mixture, mix well until smooth and pour into a greased microwave Tupperware.

3. Microwave on high for about 1 minute 30 seconds. When ready bring out the Tupperware, turn it upside down to make the bread come out easily.

4. Once cool, it can be sliced. Enjoy!

Nutrition Information Per- Serving: Calories: 136 *kcal; Fat:* 11g; *Carbohydrates:* 1.7g; *Protein:* 8.2 g

Low Carb Yeast Sandwich Bread
So fluffy and comforting. Enjoy!

Prep Time: 2 hours

Cook Time: 10 minutes

Serves: 12 slices

Ingredients

¾ cup pecan flour

¼ cup coconut flour

½ cup dark rye flour

1 cup wheat gluten, blended

1 ¼ cups water, warm

3 tablespoons butter

¾ teaspoon baking powder

¼ ginger powder

1-1/2 tablespoons yeast

½ teaspoon sugar

1 teaspoon cider vinegar

1 teaspoon cardamom

¼ cup flaxseed meal, blended

1/4 cup flax seed

1 teaspoon salt

Directions

1. Add ginger, yeast, sugar, and half of the warm water in a bowl. Mix together and set aside.

2. Add together the blended gluten, coconut flour, pecan, dark rye flour, and flaxseed meal. Mix well and set aside.

3. Add small flour mixture to the yeast mixture slowly to a stand mixer and beat on low speed for about 1 minute, and let it stand for about 10 minutes.

4. Then add cardamom, salt, and baking powder into the mixture. Melt butter and put vinegar in it, add butter mixture to dough.

5. Beat for about 1 minute until well mixed then set mixer on medium and add the remaining flour mixture to the dough.

6. Put the flaxseeds, knead for about 5 minutes, oil a bowl and place dough in it, and cover for about an hour. Then shape dough into a loaf and place in a greased loaf pan.

7. Bake in an oven for about 40 minutes at 350°F, slice when cool completely and enjoy!

Nutrition Information Per- Serving: Calories: 165kcal; Fat: 9g; Carbohydrates: 9g; Protein: 11g

BREADS ROLLS RECIPES

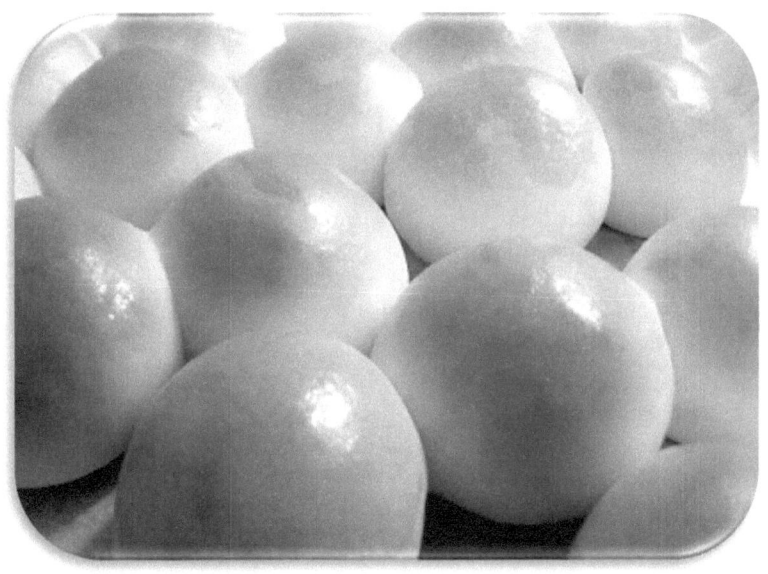

Cheddar Garlic Fathead Rolls

So delicious! You need to try this.

Prep Time: 10 minutes

Cook Time: 25 minutes

Serves: 8 rolls

Ingredients

1/2 cup coconut flour

8 ounces cheddar cheese, grated

1/4 cup protein powder, unflavored

4 teaspoon baking powder

1 teaspoon garlic powder

2 cloves garlic, minced

2 eggs

4 tablespoon butter

1 tablespoon parsley, sliced

1 egg white

Salt

Garlic Butter

Directions

1. Add cheese and 2 tablespoon of butter in a microwave bowl, let it melt for about 30 seconds. Then add protein powder, coconut flour, garlic powder, baking powder, and salt.

2. Add the eggs and egg white and knead together with a spatula. Grease you hand and roll into 8 balls and put into a baking pan.

3. Melt 2 tablespoon of butter, add parsley and garlic. Mix together and brush half of mixture on the rolls, then bake in the oven at 350°F for about 25 minutes.

4. When brown, bring out from the oven and let it cool for about 15 minutes, remove from the pan and brush with the remaining butter mixture. Enjoy!

Nutrition Information Per- Serving: Calories: 230kcal: Fat: 15.9g: Carbohydrates: 5.9g: Protein: 12.2g

Keto Bread Rolls
Satisfying tools for you.

Prep Time: 15 minutes

Cook Time: 1 hour

Serves: 6 rolls

Ingredients

3-1/3 tablespoon flax seeds, blended

1-1/4 cup almond flour

2 1/2 tsp of baking soda

1/2 cup psyllium husk powder

1-1/4 teaspoon cream

1 teaspoon salt

Water

Directions

1. Add 3 tablespoon flax seeds and water, mix together to make flax egg and set aside.

2. Add almond flour, 1/3 flax seed, baking soda, and husk powder in a bowl, add flax egg and mix with an electric mixer

3. Boil the water in a small pot, and add slowly to the mixture in the mixer. Mix until combined.

4. After 5 minutes roll dough into 6 balls, put into baking sheet with parchment paper and bake in oven at 375°Ffor about 50 minutes.

5. Let it cool completely before serving.

Nutrition Information Per- Serving: Calories: 230kcal: Fat: 14.6g: Carbohydrates: 23.6g: Protein: 6.5g

Hawaiian Sweet Rolls

This is really sweet! You will ask for more.

Prep Time: 15 minutes

Cook Time: 20 minutes

Serves: 10 rolls

Ingredients

1-1/2 cups Almond Flour

3 cups Mozzarella cheese, shredded

2 teaspoon Baking Powder

3 oz. cream cheese

3/4 cup Swerve, powdered

6 drops Pineapple oil

1 teaspoon ginger paste

2 eggs

Directions

1. Mix almond flour, swerve, and baking powder in a bowl. Melt cream cheese and Mozzarella cheese in the microwave.

2. Pour cheeses into the flour mixture, ad fresh ginger, egg, and pineapple oil. Mix well until combined.

3. Knead dough thoroughly until a bit sticky. Roll into 10 balls and place in a greased pan.

4. Bake for about 20 minutes at 425°F until brown. Let it cool completely and serve.

Nutrition Information Per- Serving: Calories: 99 kcal: Fat: 4.1g: Carbohydrates: 2.8g: Protein: 12.7g

Keto Dinner Rolls
Delicious and tasty rolls. Try it!

Prep Time: 10 minutes

Cook Time: 12 minutes

Serves: 8 rolls

Ingredients

1-1/2 cup almond flour

1 tablespoon baking powder

2 tablespoon protein powder, unflavored

2-1/2 cup Mozzarella cheese, shredded

1 tablespoon Erythritol

3 tablespoon butter divided

21/4 teaspoon dry yeast

3 eggs, beaten

Directions

1. Mix almond flour, baking powder, Erythritol, protein powder, and yeast together in a bowl and put aside.

2. Melt shredded Mozzarella cheese and butter in a microwave for about 30 seconds and add to the mixture that was set aside.

3. Mix dough well and form into 8 balls, place rolls in an oiled skillet with parchment paper

4. Brush with egg, and bake in the oven for about 12 mins at 400°F. When ready brush with some butter and serve! Enjoy!

Nutrition Information Per- Serving: Calories: 150kcal: Fat: 7.9g: Carbohydrates: 4.9g: Protein: 14.7g

Keto Fiber Bread Rolls

So fluffy and delicious. This is for you!

Prep Time: 10 minutes

Cook Time: 40 minutes

Serves: 11 rolls

Ingredients

1 cup Almond Flour

4tsp baking Powder

3tablespoon Psyllium Husk

3/4 Cup oat Fiber

4 Tablespoon Oil

2 tablespoon Vinegar

1 oz Protein Powder

1 teaspoon salt

2 tablespoon Water

1 Cup Yogurt

4 Eggs

Directions

1. Add Almond Flour, baking Powder, Protein Powder, and psyllium husk in a bowl. Mix well until combine.

2. Whisk eggs, and add to the flour mixture, add Yogurt, Vinegar, water, oil and salt. Cover for about 30 minutes.

3. Then make 11 rolls with the dough and place in a baking sheet with Parchment paper, sprinkle oat fiber and bake in an oven for about 40 minutes 300F. Enjoy!

Nutrition Information Per- Serving: Calories: 177 kcal: Fat: 14g: Carbohydrates: 7g: Protein: 11g

BUNS RECIPES

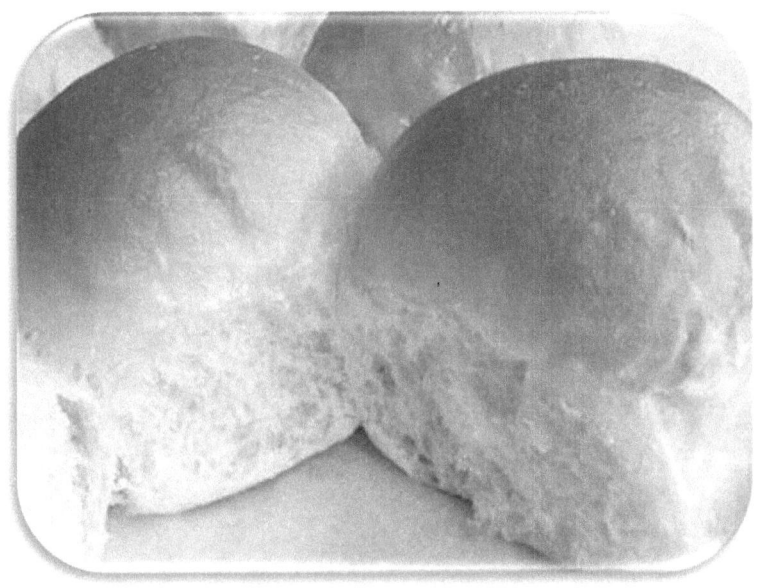

Keto Bread Buns

So tasty and irresistible!

Prep Time: 5 minutes

Cook Time: 50 minutes

Serves: 9

Ingredients

1 1/4 cups almond flour

1 cup boiling water

2 teaspoon vinegar

1 tablespoon sesame seeds

5 tablespoon psyllium husks, grounded

2 teaspoon baking powder

1 tablespoon olive oil

1 teaspoon salt

3 egg whites

Directions

1. Mix well in a bowl almond flour, baking powder, psyllium husk, and salt.

2. Add vinegar and egg whites. Use electric mixer to mix slowly and add water.

3. When combined, make 9 buns with the dough and put them on a baking sheet, brush with oil and sprinkle sesame seeds on it.

4. Bake for about 50 minutes at 350F. Serve and enjoy!

Nutrition Information Per- Serving: Calories: 105kcal: Fat: 7g: Carbohydrates: 2g: Protein: 9g

Keto Burger Buns
Tasty and comforting buns for you

Prep Time: 15 minutes

Cook Time: 25 minutes

Serves: 8

Ingredients

1 1/2 cup Almond Flour,

1 teaspoon Baking Powder

1 tablespoon Coconut Flour

1/2 cup Chorizo, diced

1 teaspoon baking Soda

1 tablespoon Flax Meal

1/4 teaspoon Real Salt

1 tablespoon Vinegar

1 tablespoon Sesame Seeds

5 eggs

Directions

1. Mix together in a bowl coconut flour, almond flour, baking powder, baking soda, flax seeds and salt.

2. Put vinegar, egg, and chorizo, then mix well. Use a spoon to fill the dough into a greased pudding tin.

3. Sprinkle on them sesame seeds and put to oven to bake for about 25 minutes at 350 F.

4. Let buns cool completely and serve.

Nutrition Information Per- Serving: Calories: 296kcal: Fat: 22.4g: Carbohydrates: 6.4g: Protein: 15.4g

Dark Bread Buns
Easy and crunchy buns. So healthy!

Prep Time: 10 minutes

Cook Time: 20 minutes

Serves: 8

Ingredients

½ cup coconut flour

¼ cups psyllium husk powder

½ cup black sesame seeds, crushed

20g potato fiber, blended

3.5 ounce ground flaxseed

11/4 cup hot water

5 tsp yeast

3 tbsp vinegar

1 tsp baking soda

11/2 tsp cumin

4 egg whites

1 tsp salt

Directions

1. Mix together coconut flour, psyllium husk powder, potato fiber, ground flaxseed, yeast, and baking soda.

2. Put apple cider vinegar and egg whites. Add hot water and mix to combine.

3. Compress them into 8 buns and garnish with sesame seeds. Bake for about 30 minutes at 200C in the oven. Enjoy hot or cold.

Nutrition Information Per- Serving: Calories: 195 kcal: Fat: 15g: Carbohydrates: 1,6g: Protein: 8g

Low Carb Cauliflower Burger Buns
So sweet and irresistible. Try it.

Prep Time: 10 minutes

Cook Time: 25 minutes

Serves: 8

Ingredients

¼ cup almond flour

¼ cup coconut flour

1/2 teaspoon baking powder

1/4 teaspoon seasoning

2 cups cauliflower, riced

¼ cup parmesan, grated

½ cup cheese, grated

1 teaspoon dried chives, chopped

Sesame seeds

1/4 teaspoon salt

2 eggs

Directions

1. Add almond flour, coconut flour, baking powder, seasoning, cauliflower, parmesan, cheese, chives, eggs, and salt. Use a mixer to mix well.

2. Use your hands to knead until a bit sticky, then make 8 buns and place on a greased baking pan.

3. Sprinkle sesame seeds on the buns and bake for about 25 minutes at 200°C. Enjoy!

Nutrition Information Per- Serving: Calories: 95kcal: Fat: 6g: Carbohydrates: 2g: Protein: 6g

Perfect Keto Buns

So tasty and yummy. Really perfect for you!

Prep Time: 5 minutes

Cook Time: 15 minutes

Serves: 5

Ingredients

4 tablespoon almond flour

1/4 tsp xanthan gum

1 tablespoon parmesan cheese

1 cup cheddar cheese

3 eggs, beaten

Salt

Directions

1. In a bowl, put eggs, almond flour, xanthan gum, parmesan cheese, cheddar cheese, and salt.

2. Mix to combine and make 5 buns of desired shape and place in a baking sheet with parchment paper.

3. Bake for about 12 minutes or more if not ready at 350 degrees, then broil for about 3 minutes. Enjoy!

Nutrition Information Per- Serving: Calories: 118.2*kcal: Fat:* 10.2g: *Carbohydrates:* 0.4g: *Protein:* 7.2g

BAGEL RECIPES

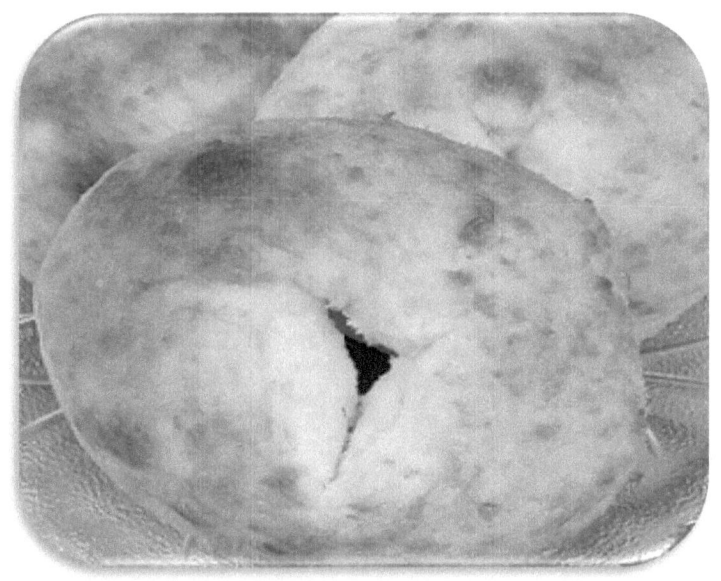

Keto Fathead Bagels

So comforting you will like this

Prep Time: 10 minutes

Cook Time: 20 minutes

Serves: 4

Ingredients

1 cup almond flour

1 1/2 cups mozzarella cheese, shredded

2 tablespoons cream cheese

1 tablespoon dry onion, minced

1 1/2 teaspoons baking powder

2 teaspoons white sesame seeds

2 teaspoons poppy seeds

1/2 tablespoon olive oil

1/4 teaspoon salt

Seasoning mix

1 egg

Directions

1. Pour all seasoning mix in a bowl and stir well, in another bowl put almond flour, baking powder, and some of the seasoning mix. Mix to combine.
2. Add cream cheese and mozzarella cheese, microwave for about 1 minutes, stir and microwave until the cheese is melted.

3. Add eggs, stir well and knead with your hands until smooth, make 4 rolls with the dough, and place them on a baking sheet lined with parchment paper.

4. Brush with oil and sprinkle left over seasoning mix on top and bake for about 20 minutes at 375 F. Enjoy!

Nutrition Information Per- Serving: Calories: 370kcal: Fat: 30g: Carbohydrates: 10g: Protein: 19g

Bagel Buns With Yeast
Sweet buns with comforting taste.

Prep Time: 1 hour 10 minutes

Cook Time: 25 minutes

Serves: 12

Ingredients

3/4 cup Coconut Flour

1 teaspoon baking powder

2 teaspoon Chicory Root

1/2 cup warm water

8 oz. Mozzarella cheese, shredded

1/2 teaspoon Xanthan Gum

1/4 teaspoon Salt

2 ¼ teaspoon Yeast

2 eggs, beaten

Directions

1. Put water in a bowl, add yeast and chicory root. Put aside for about 10 minutes.

2. In a bowl put Coconut flour, baking powder, Xanthan gum and salt. Stir to combine.

3. Melt shredded cheese in a microwave, add eggs to it and mix well. Pour into the flour mixture and add the yeast mixture.

4. Knead with hands until dough is a bit sticky and cover with a towel. Set aside and hour.

5. Make dough into 12 pieces and bake for about 24 minutes at 110 degrees.

Nutrition Information Per- Serving: Calories: 106kcal: Fat: 6g: Carbohydrates: 6g: Protein: 8g

Low-Carb Multi Seed Bagels

Fluffy and healthy bagels. So tasty

Prep Time: 10 minutes

Cook Time: 20 minutes

Serves: 12

Ingredients

1 cup coconut flour

1 tablespoon baking powder

½ cup sesame seeds

½ cup pumpkin seeds

1 teaspoon Celtic sea salt

¼ cup Psyllium Fiber

½ cup hemp hearts

1 cup warm water

6 egg whites, blended

Directions

1. In a bowl, put coconut flour, baking powder, Psyllium Fiber, hemp hearts, and Celtic sea, mix well to combine.

2. Add egg whites, knead well with hands, put water and mix until dough is smooth.

3. Make 6 rolls from dough, place on a baking sheet with parchment paper, and shape into bagel of your choice.

4. Sprinkle on top sesame seeds and pumpkin seeds and bake for about 55 minutes at 350F.

Nutrition Information Per- Serving: Calories: 352kcal: Fat: 19g: Carbohydrates: 8g: Protein: 18g

Low Carb Cinnamon Sugar Bagels

Soft and doughy bagels for you.

Prep Time: 15 minutes

Cook Time: 25 minutes

Serves: 6

Ingredients

1 3/4 cups almond flour

1/4 cup coconut flour

2 1/2 cups mozzarella, shredded

1 teaspoon baking soda

1 tablespoon cinnamon, divided

2 teaspoon cream of tartar

2 1/2 cups mozzarella, shredded

3 tablespoon sweetener

2 oz. cream chees

3 eggs, beaten

Directions

1. Put almond flour, baking soda, coconut flour, 1 tablespoon sweetener, cream of tartar, and 1 tablespoon cinnamon in a bowl. Mix well.

2. Microwave mozzarella and cream cheese for about 60 seconds. Stir and add to the first flour mixture.

3. Add egg and knead with your hands to form smooth dough. Make 6 rolls with dough and place on a baking sheet with parchment paper.

4. Shape bagels as desired and brush with egg. Add remaining sweetener and cinnamon together and sprinkle on top. Bake for about 14 minutes at 400 degrees. Enjoy bagels!

Nutrition Information Per- Serving: Calories: 317 kcal: Fat: 19.9g: Carbohydrates: 17.8g: Protein: 25.4g

Flavored Bagels
Tasty and well flavored bagels for you.

Prep Time: 15 minutes

Cook Time: 20 minutes

Serves: 8

Ingredients

6 ounces almond flour

2 teaspoons baking powder

10 ounces mozzarella, melted

2 tablespoons butter, melted

1 teaspoon Chicory Root

2 tablespoons warm water

1 teaspoon xanthan gum

2 tablespoons seasoning

2 teaspoons yeast

3 eggs

Directions

1. Mix yeast and chicory root inn warm water and set aside. When yeast is foamy, add almond flour, xanthan gum, and baking powder.

2. Mix well and put melted cheese and mozzarella, 2 eggs, and mix until smooth dough forms.

3. Knead with hands thoroughly and make 8 rolls from dough. Place rolls on a baking sheet with parchment paper and shape as desired.

4. Beat the remaining egg, brush the bagels with the egg, seasoning the bagels, and set aside for about 15 minutes. Set oven to 355F and bake for about 20 minutes. Enjoy when ready.

Nutrition Information Per- Serving: Calories: 292kcal: Fat: 23g: Carbohydrates: 7.5g: Protein: 15g

PIZZA DOUGH RECIPES

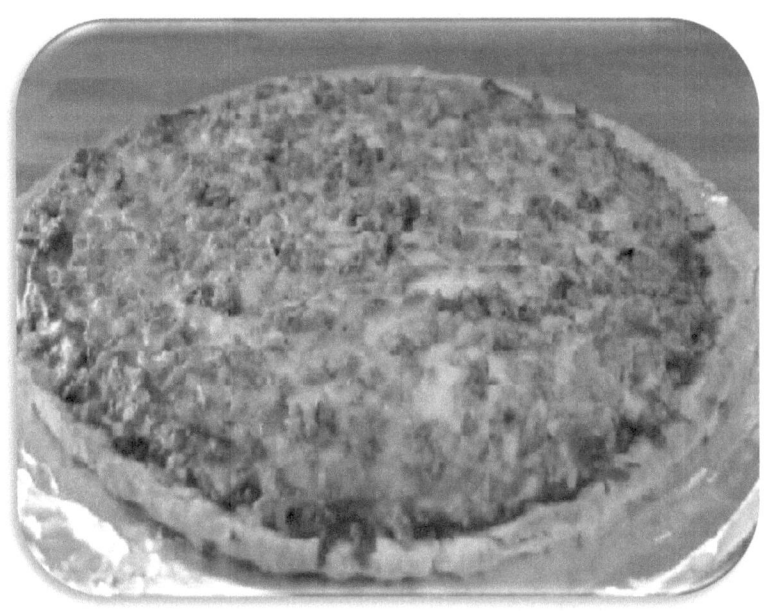

Keto Fathead Pizza Doug

So tasty! You will enjoy it

Prep Time: 15 minutes

Cook Time: 20 minutes

Serves: 4

Ingredients

3/4 cup almond flour

2 tablespoon cream cheese, softened

1 3/4 cup mozzarella, shredded

1/2 teaspoon garlic powder

1/2 teaspoon seasoning

1/4 teaspoon pepper

1/4 teaspoon salt

1 egg, beaten

Pizza toppings, as desired

Directions

1. Put in a microwave for about 1 minute; almond flour, cream cheese, and mozzarella cheese.

2. Mix to combine and put the egg and seasoning, stir and knead with your hands.

3. Divide into 4 pieces and flatten with a rolling pin and give a desired shape.

4. Put your desired toppings and bake for about 15 minutes at 425F. Enjoy!

Nutrition Information Per- Serving: Calories: 300kcal: Fat: 22.5g: Carbohydrates: 4g: Protein: 20.5g

Yeast Pizza Dough
Very easy and tasty. Yummy!

Prep Time: 30 minutes

Cook Time: 10 minutes

Serves: 1 crust

Ingredients

1½ cups Almond Flour

¼ teaspoon Baking Powder

1¼ teaspoon Xanthan Gum

1 tablespoon Yeast

½ tablespoon Vinegar

1 tablespoon Yeast

¼ cup Warm Water

2 egg whites

1 egg

1 teaspoon salt

Directions

1. Add yeast to warm water and set aside to proof, mix Almond Flour, baking powder, Xanthan gum and salt together. Mix well to combine.

2. Mix eggs and vinegar with a mixer, add half of the flour mixture and the yeast mixture to the mixer, mix well and add the remaining half of the flour mixture.

3. Put the dough on a pizza pan with parchment and press it to make it flat. Cover with a towel for about 15 minutes to rise.

4. Bake for about 10 minutes at 375F, then add pizza toppings and bake for few minutes. Enjoy!

Nutrition Information Per- Serving: Calories: 180 kcal: Fat: 15g: Carbohydrates: 7g: Protein: 8g

Bacon Fathead Pizza Dough
Comforting and tasty. You will like it.

Prep Time: 20 minutes

Cook Time: 40 minutes

Serves: 6

Ingredients

1 cup Almond flour

1/2 tablespoon garlic powder

3 teaspoon Tomato paste

3 cups Mozzarella, melted

1/3 cup Tomatoes, sliced

1/4 cup Olives

1/2 cup Bacon

1 egg

Directions

1. Add almond flour, garlic powder, and 2 cups mozzarella, Knead with your hands. Put egg and mix well to combine.

2. Put dough on the greased baking pan and use spatula to press down to make it flat, bake for about 10 minutes at 390F.

3. After 10 minutes spread on top tomato paste, put bacon, tomatoes, shredded cheese, and olives. Then bake for another 10 minutes. It's ready.

Nutrition Information Per- Serving: Calories: 312kcal: Fat: 24g: Carbohydrates: 5g: Protein: 23g

Low carb Fathead Pizza Dough
Delicious! You will ask for more.

Prep Time: 15 minutes

Cook Time: 15 minutes

Serves: 6

Ingredients

3/4 cup almond flour

2 cups mozzarella, shredded

3 tablespoon tomato sauce

1/4 red pepper, chopped

1 teaspoon oregano

12 slices pepperoni

2 oz. cream cheese

1 egg, beaten

Directions

1. Microwave 1 1\2 mozzarella cheese, almond flour, and cream cheese for about 90 seconds and stir.

2. Add egg and knead with your hand to form smooth dough, put on a baking sheet with parchment paper and roll with a rolling pin. Use fork to make holes.

3. Bake for about 10 minutes at 425F. Then spread on the top tomato sauce, cheese, pepperoni slices, and red pepper. Bake for about 5 minutes and enjoy!

Nutrition Information Per- Serving: Calories: 243kcal: Fat: 19g: Carbohydrates: 4g: Protein: 12g

Fat Head Pizza Dough

This classic pizza is healthy and satisfying. Let's bake!

Prep Time: 5 minutes

Cook Time: 15 minutes

Serves: 4

Ingredients

1/2 cup almond flour

1.5 cups mozzarella cheese, {shredded and melted}

1 tablespoon seasoning {Italian or any of your choice}

Toppings {as desired}

1 egg

Directions

1. Add almond flour, mozzarella cheese, and egg.

2. Mix well to combine and put seasoning.

3. Mix well to combine, and put on the baking sheet with parchment paper and knead with your hands.

4. Use fork to make holes on crust, bake for about 8 minutes at 425 degrees, and add toppings.

5. Bake for about 10 minutes and enjoy.

Nutrition Information Per- Serving: Calories: 229 kcal: Fat: 18.1g: Carbohydrates: 3.5g: Protein: 13.9g

TORTILLA RECIPES

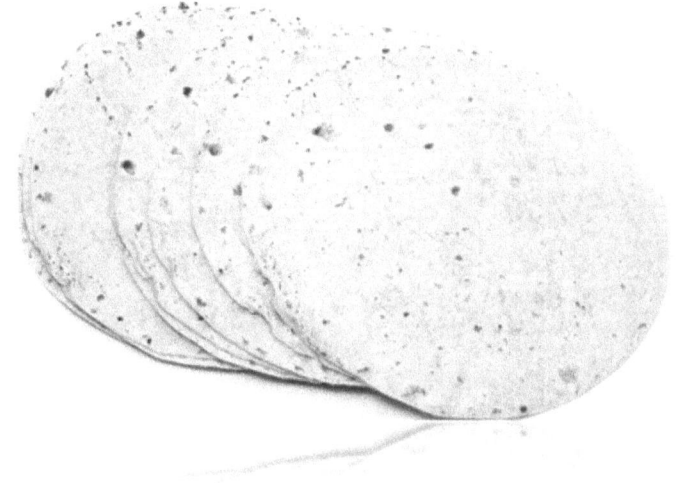

Keto Coconut Flour Tortillas

Easy and tasty.

Prep Time: 10 minutes

Cook Time: 8 minutes

Serves: 4

Ingredients

5 tablespoon coconut flour

1/2 teaspoon xanthan gum

1/2 teaspoon baking powder

2 tablespoon water

1/4 teaspoon salt

1 egg, beaten

Directions

1. Put in a bowl coconut flour, xanthan gum, baking powder, and salt. Mix well to combine.

2. Add 1 tablespoon water and egg, mix until a smooth dough forms. If too thick add more water

3. Then cut into 4 pieces, use a rolling pin to press each tortilla.

4. Heat up a skillet on high heat, and cook each tortilla for about 45 seconds.

5. When bubbles and puffs appears it's ready. Enjoy!

Nutrition Information Per- Serving: Calories: 54kcal: Fat: 18g: Carbohydrates: 5g: Protein: 2g

Easy Low Carb Tortilla

Satisfying and super easy. Try it!

Prep Time: 5 minutes

Cook Time: 30 minutes

Serves: 12

Ingredients

3 tablespoon psyllium husk powder

1 cup coconut flour

1/2 teaspoon baking powder

1 teaspoon garlic powder

4 tablespoon coconut oil

3 cups hot water

1 teaspoon salt

Directions

1. Mix coconut flour, psyllium husk powder, garlic powder, baking powder and salt together in bowl.

2. Add coconut oil, water as needed, mix and keep for about 20 minutes until it absorb the liquids.

3. Cut dough into 12 slices, use a rolling pin and a parchment paper if sticky to press to a desired flat size.

4. Heat a skillet or non-stick pan on medium heat, put some coconut nut oil in and cook tortilla one after the other for about 60 seconds, or depending on the pan size.

5. Enjoy!

Nutrition Information Per- Serving: Calories: 89*kcal: Fat:* 5g: *Carbohydrates:* 7g: *Protein:* 1g

Smoked Paprika Tortilla

*Comforting and tasty to your satis*faction.

Prep Time: 5 minutes

Cook Time: 5 minutes

Serves: 4

<u>Ingredients</u>

1/4 Cup Coconut Flour

1 Cup Egg Whites

1/2 tsp Smoked Paprika

1/2 teaspoon cumin

1 cup water

<u>Directions</u>

1. Mix coconut flour, egg whites, and water together.

2. Put cumin, and smoked paprika, mix well to combine.

3. On high heat, heat a frying pan, pour a little portion of coconut oil, and put enough flour mixture. Cook like a very tin pan cakes.

4. When bubbling, flip tortilla onto the other side and cook for about 30 seconds. If flour mixture remains, do the same.

Nutrition Information Per- Serving: Calories: 71*kcal: Fat:* 2g: *Carbohydrates:* 2.5g: *Protein:* 8g

Keto Vegan Tortilla

Tasty and filling!

Prep Time: 5 minutes

Cook Time: 5 minutes

Serves: 1

Ingredients

2 tablespoons almond flour

1 teaspoon psyllium husk powder

1 teaspoon chia seeds

3 tablespoons water

Salt

Directions

1. Mix almond flour, psyllium husk powder, chia seeds, and salt.

2. Put water and stir, to form a smooth dough and place on a microwave plate.

3. Bake for about 5 minutes at 500 watts. Enjoy when cool.

Nutrition Information Per- Serving: Calories: 127.4kcal: Fat: 8.4g: Carbohydrates: 10.7g: Protein: 3.9g

Pork Rind Tortillas

So satisfying and yummy! You need this.

Prep Time: 5 minutes

Cook Time: 15 minutes

Serves: 12

Ingredients

4 oz. Pork Rinds

8 oz. cream cheese

1 tablespoon Cumin, powdered

1/3 cup Water

1 teaspoon Salt

8 eggs

Directions

1. Blitz pork rinds in a food processor for about 10 seconds, and put cheese, eggs, cumin, water, and salt. Blitz for about 45 seconds.

2. Put a non-stick pan on the stove on high heat and add a little oil. Add a little portion of batter (blitzed ingredients} and spread with spatula like a pan cake on the pan.

3. Cook for about 2 minutes or until brown, flip tortilla too when brown. Add more batter and follow the same procedure.

Nutrition Information Per- Serving: Calories: 168.5kcal: Fat: 12.4g: Carbohydrates: 0.9g: Protein: 11.4g

MUFFINS RECIPES

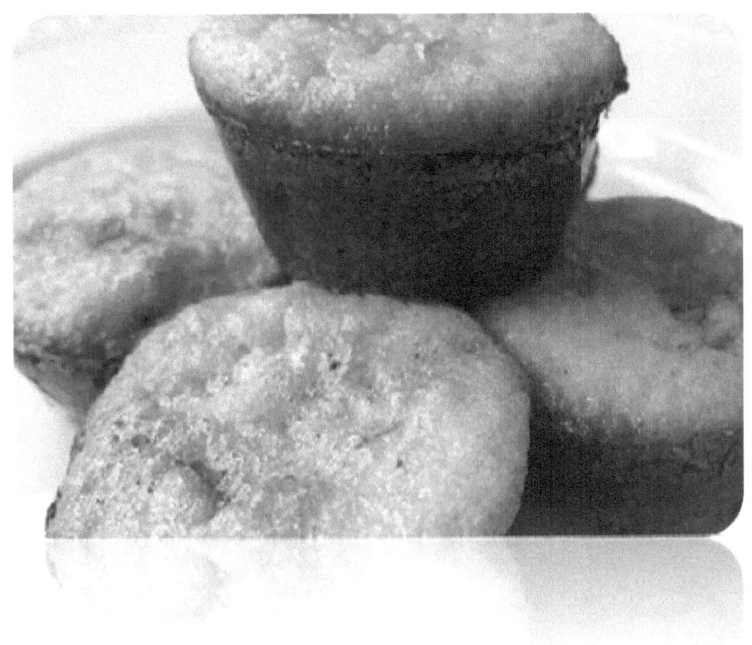

Keto Blueberry Muffins

Just a bite, will tell you how tasty it is.

Prep Time: 10 minutes

Cook Time: 20 minutes

Serves: 12

Ingredients

1 1/4 cups almond flour

3/4 teaspoon baking soda

1 cup blueberries

1/2 cup almond butter

2 teaspoon vanilla extract

2 tablespoon milk

1/2 cup erythritol

1 tablespoon lemon juice

3 eggs

Directions

1. Mix together almond butter, almond flour, erythritol, baking soda, milk, vanilla, lemon juice, the eggs and salt.

2. Mix to combine and put 2/3 of the blueberries, and line a 12 cup muffin pan with parchment liners.

3. Put mixture into each cups and bake for about 20 minutes at 325. Once cool enjoy!

Nutrition Information Per- Serving: Calories: 156kcal: Fat: 12g: Carbohydrates: 6g: Protein: 6g

Ham And Zucchini Muffins

Fluffy and well flavored. For you

Prep Time: 10 minutes

Cook Time: 35 minutes

Serves: 12

Ingredients

1 cup almond flour

1 teaspoon baking powder

1/3 cup sour cream

100g cheese, grated

1 zucchini, grated

150g ham, diced

1/2 teaspoon salt

1/2 teaspoon pepper

4 eggs

Directions

1. Mix sour cream, cheese, zucchini, ham, and eggs in a bowl.

2. Mix well almond flour, pepper, baking powder, and salt in another bowl. Then pour the first mixture in.

3. Mix well and put into a 12 cup muffin tin and bake for about 40 minutes in the oven at 356F.

4. Let it cool before serving. Enjoy!

Nutrition Information Per- Serving: Calories: 135*kcal: Fat:* 9g: *Carbohydrates:* 3g: *Protein:* 9g

Almond Flour Banana Muffins
This is Healthy and filling.

Prep Time: 10 minutes

Cook Time: 30 minutes

Serves: 12

Ingredients

3 cups almond flour

1/2 teaspoon baking powder

1 teaspoon baking soda

3 ripe bananas

1 teaspoon vanilla extract

1/4 cup dark chocolate chips

1 teaspoon cinnamon

1/4 teaspoon salt

3 eggs

Directions

1. Blend bananas, cinnamon, vanilla, baking powder, baking soda, eggs, and salt together.

2. Add almond flour and chocolate chips to it and stir using a spatula. Pour into a 12 cup muffin tin.

3. Bake for about 30 minutes at 350 degrees in the oven. Make sure its golden brown and cool before serving.

Nutrition Information Per- Serving: Calories: 214kcal: Fat: 6.7g: Carbohydrates: 13.6g: Protein: 6g

Low Carb Pumpkin Muffins
So delicious and super easy. Let's bake.

Prep Time: 5 minutes

Cook Time: 18 minutes

Serves: 7

Ingredients

3/4 tablespoon stevia powder

1/4 teaspoon cardamom powder

1 teaspoon baking powder

1/4 teaspoon baking soda

1/2 cup pumpkin puree

1/2 cup unsweetened almond butter

1/2 teaspoon cinnamon

1/4 teaspoon ground ginger

1/4 teaspoon ground cloves

2 tablespoon oil

4 eggs

Directions

1. Mix well stevia powder, cardamom powder, baking powder, baking soda, pumpkin puree, almond butter, cinnamon, ground ginger, ground cloves, oil, and eggs in a bowl.

2. Pour in into 7 muffin cups and bake for about 18 minutes at 375F. Let it cool before serving. Enjoy!

Nutrition Information Per- Serving: Calories: 185kcal: Fat: 15.83g: Carbohydrates: 5.99g: Protein: 7.74g

Cheese Muffins

Cheesy, fluffy, and super delicious. You will enjoy it.

Prep Time: 10 minutes

Cook Time: 35 minutes

Serves: 12

Ingredients

1 cup Almond Flour

2 teaspoons Baking Powder

1/2 cup cheddar cheese, grated

1/4 cup Heavy Whipping Cream

1/2 teaspoon granulated garlic

1/2 cup Black Chia Seeds

1/4 cup butter, melted

4 eggs

Directions

1. Mix together almond flour, baking powder, granulated garlic, eggs, and chia seeds.

2. Add butter, cheese and heavy whipping cream. Pour into a 12 cup muffin tin.

3. Bake for about 40 minutes at 350F, until golden brown. Let it cool before serving.

Nutrition Information Per- Serving: Calories: 182kcal: Fat: 15g: Carbohydrates: 5g: Protein: 6g

CRACKER RECIPES

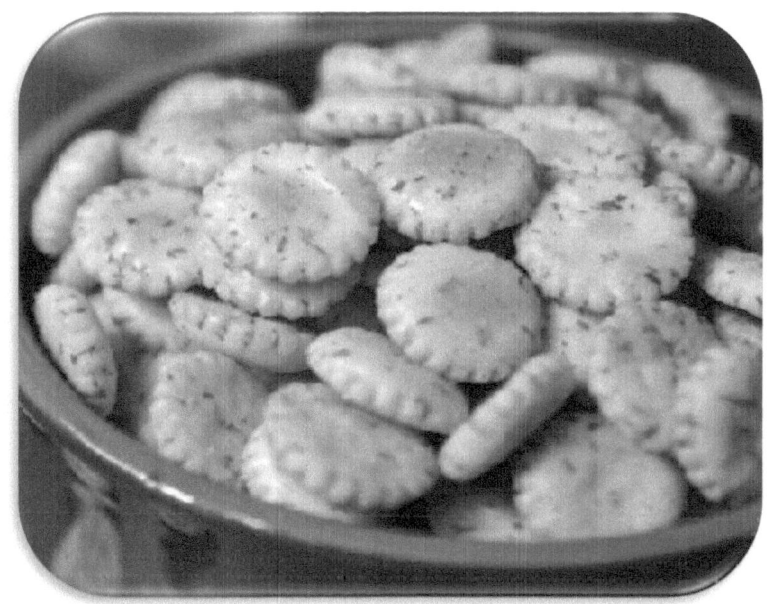

Low Carb Jalapeño Cheese Crackers

Crispy and yummy!

Prep Time: 5 minutes

Cook Time: 15 minutes

Serves: 16

Ingredients

4 jalapeno peppers, sliced

1 pound cheddar cheese, sliced

Directions

1. Put sliced cheese on baking sheet lined with parchment, and garnish with jalapeno peppers.

2. Bake for about 15 minutes at 425F, remove when it's a bit brown.

3. Enjoy when completely cool.

Nutrition Information Per- Serving: Calories: 106kcal: Fat: 9g: Carbohydrates: 1g: Protein: 7g

Easy Crackers

Healthy crackers for you. Very easy!

Prep Time: 10 minutes

Cook Time: 40 minutes

Serves: 10

Ingredients

2 tablespoon Almond flour

1/4 teaspoon cayenne pepper powder

1/4 teaspoon hot curry powder

1 tablespoon chopped walnuts

1/4 cup Sunflower seeds

1/2 cup Chia seeds

1/4 cup Pumpkin seeds

1/4 cup Flax seeds

1 1/2 cups hot water

Salt

Directions

1. Mix together Almond flour, cayenne pepper powder, and curry powder in a bowl.

2. Add walnuts, Sunflower seeds, Chia seeds, Pumpkin seeds, and Flax seeds.

3. Put hot water and stir well to combine. Put on a well- greased baking sheet and spread.

4. Use knife to mark some lines on the layer, to make it easy to break. Bake for about 70 minutes at 350F. Enjoy when cool.

Nutrition Information Per- Serving: Calories: 97.3kcal: Fat: 6.1g: Carbohydrates: 7.9g: Protein: 4.5g

Keto Rosemary Crackers
Low carb tasty cracker. You need to try this.

Prep Time: 5 minutes

Cook Time: 25 minutes

Serves: 40

Ingredients

¼ cup coconut flour

10g hemp flour

¾ cup organic flour

1 tablespoon rosemary, chopped

3 tbsp dark chia seeds

1 tbsp ground flaxseed

2 tbsp sunflower seeds

2 tbsp olive oil

1/8 cup oat bran

½ cup water

Directions

1. Mix coconut flour, hemp flour, organic flour, rosemary, dark chia seeds, flaxseed, and sunflower seeds together in a bowl.

2. Put water, oil, and keep aside for about 5 minutes.

3. Put dough on a sheet of parchment paper, and make it flat with hand. Use a rolling pin on dough to flatten more.

4. Place on a baking pan, to make it easy to break use knife to mark some lines on the dough, and bake for about 25 minutes at 180°C.

5. Serve when cool.

Nutrition Information Per- Serving: Calories: 1163kcal: Fat: 71g: Carbohydrates: 28g: Protein: 58g

Keto Goldfish Crackers
Tasty and nourishing! You will love it.

Prep Time: 10 minutes

Cook Time: 4 minutes

Serves: 2

Ingredients

1 cup Cheddar cheese

Directions

1. Cut Cheddar cheese as desired, put on a baking sheet, and keep it for 4 days to dry.

2. When hard, bake for about 4 minutes at 392F. Enjoy!

Nutrition Information Per- Serving: Calories: 203kcal: Fat: 17g: Carbohydrates: 1g: Protein: 12g

Tasty Crackers
Sumptuous! Let's bake.

Prep Time: 20 minutes

Cook Time: 30 minutes

Serves: 36

Ingredients

1 3/4 cups almond flour

1/2 teaspoon garlic powder

2 tablespoons Seasonings

1/2 teaspoon onion powder

1/4 teaspoon salt

1 egg, beaten

Directions

1. Mix egg, onion powder, garlic powder, salt, and 1 tablespoon seasoning together.

2. Add the almond flour and mix to combine. Flatten between two sheets of parchment paper.

3. Sprinkle on the dough the remaining seasoning, use a pizza cutter, and put on baking sheet.

4. Bake for about 10 minutes at 350F.

Nutrition Information Per- Serving: Calories: 212kcal: Fat: 17.1g: Carbohydrates: 5.8g: Protein: 8.1g

BREADSTICKS RECIPES

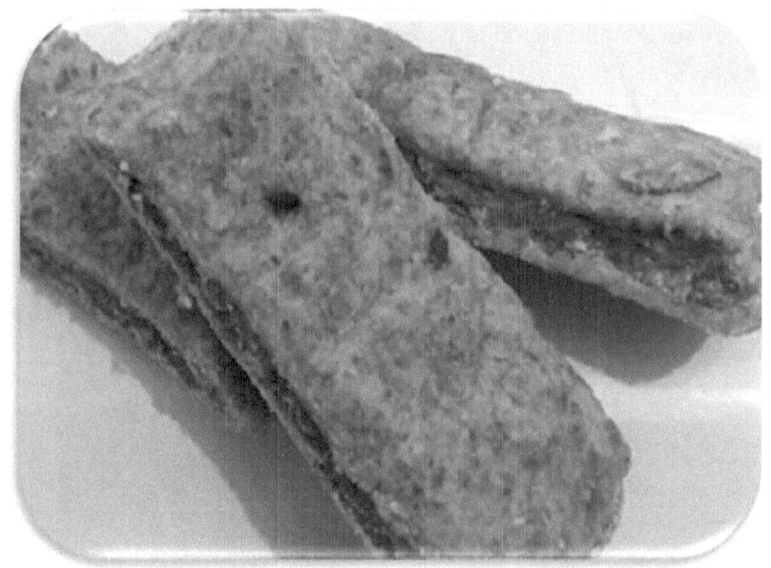

Cauliflower Breadsticks

Rich breadstick that you will like.

Prep Time: 20 minutes

Cook Time: 17 minutes

Serves: 3

Ingredients

4 ounce Almonds ground

1 cup Cauliflower rice

2 tablespoon Sesame seeds, hulled and dried

1 tablespoon Parmesan cheese, grated

½ cup Cheddar cheese, grated

1 teaspoon Italian Seasoning

1 teaspoon Oregano, dried

¼ teaspoon Black Pepper

¼ teaspoon salt

1 egg

Directions

1. Cook cauliflower rice with 1 tablespoon water for about 2 minutes and set aside to cool.

2. Put cauliflower in a food processor with ground almonds, Parmesan, cheddar, oregano, salt, Italian seasoning, and half sesame seed.

3. Let it combine well, then add egg and blend. Put in a bowl and refrigerate for about 10 minutes.

4. Put in a tray with baking paper and divide into 9 portions, roll each portion into sausage shapes and sprinkle the remaining sesame seed on it.

5. Arrange in the lined oven tray and bake for about 15 minutes at 400F.

Nutrition Information Per- Serving: Calories: 391.4kcal: Fat: 33.4g: Carbohydrates: 9.0g: Protein: 18.3g

Taco Stuffed Breadsticks
Wow! You will bake more.

Prep Time: 20 minutes

Cook Time: 17 minutes

Serves: 5

Ingredients

3/4 cup almond flour

1 3/4 cups mozzarella cheese

1 cup Mexican blend cheese, shredded

3/4 pound taco seasoned meat, cooked

2 tablespoons cream cheese

1/2 teaspoon cumin

1/4 teaspoon salt

1 egg

Directions

1. Microwave almond flour, mozzarella cheese, and cream cheese for about 30 seconds.

2. Add cumin, salt, and egg, mix to combine and knead with a rolling pin.

3. Divide into 5 portions, sprinkle shredded cheese and seasoned meat on each dough, and roll into sausage.

4. Put on baking sheet and bake for about 14 minutes. Enjoy!

Nutrition Information Per- Serving: Calories: 407 kcal: Fat: 13g: Carbohydrates: 4g: Protein: 23g

Cheesy Zucchini Breadsticks
Cheesy any tasty for you.

Prep Time: 10 minutes

Cook Time: 25 minutes

Serves: 4

Ingredients

1 tablespoon almond flour

1 zucchini, shredded and grated

1/2 cup cheddar cheese, shredded

1 cup mozzarella cheese

1 tablespoon oregano

Coriander chopped

2 eggs

Salt

Pepper

Directions

1. Mix zucchini, almond flour, mozzarella cheese, and oregano together in a bowl.

2. Spread mixture in a baking dish covered with waxed paper, roll well and bake for about 20 minutes at 350°F.

3. Sprinkle chopped coriander and cheddar cheese on it and bake for another 5 minutes.

4. When golden, it's ready.

Nutrition Information Per- Serving: Calories: 199 kcal: Fat: 14.2g: Carbohydrates: 4.7g: Protein: 14.2g

Low Carb Cauliflower Breadsticks
Well flavored and it's yummy.

Prep Time: 15 minutes

Cook Time: 15 minutes

Serves: 5

Ingredients

1 cup Mozzarella cheese, shredded

1/2 cup Parmesan cheese, shaved

1/2 tablespoon basil, chopped

1/2 tablespoon parsley, chopped

1/2 teaspoon ground black pepper

1/2 tablespoon garlic, minced

1 cauliflower, riced

1 teaspoon salt

1 egg

Directions

1. Put cauliflower in a food processor to make it moist, add 1/2 cup Mozzarella cheese, egg, basil, garlic, Parmesan cheese, parsley, black pepper, and salt.

2. Mix well to combine and place into the baking sheet lined with parchment paper, spread well.

3. Bake for about 12 minutes in an oven at 425°F, take out from oven and sprinkle the remaining Mozzarella cheese on it. Bake for about 10 minutes and cut into breadsticks. Enjoy!

Nutrition Information Per- Serving: Calories: 143kcal: Fat: 9g: Carbohydrates: 2g: Protein: 11g

Breadsticks With Sesame Seeds

Yummy! This will be your favorite.

Prep Time: 10 minutes

Cook Time: 15 minutes

Serves: 12

Ingredients

¾ cup almond flour

1½ cups mozzarella cheese, grated

1 tablespoon Sesame seeds

2 tablespoon cream cheese

3 tablespoon butter, melted

¼ teaspoon salt

Directions

1. Microwave cream and mozzarella cheese together in a bowl for about 2 minutes.

2. Add to the melted cheese almond flour and salt. Mix well and place on a parchment paper and knead with your hands to make it flat.

3. Cut into 12, and form into breadsticks. Put them in a tray lined with parchment paper and brush with butter.

4. Sprinkle sesame seeds on top and bake for about 15 minutes at 400°F until brown. Enjoy!

Nutrition Information Per- Serving: Calories: 90kcal: Fat: 11g: Carbohydrates: 1g: Protein: 5g